Turpentine
as
Medicine?

The Medicinal Healing
Benefits of Terpenic Oil

Ryder Management Inc.

Epigraph

"It is easy to get a thousand prescriptions but hard to get one single remedy."
Chinese Proverb

"He's the best physician that knows the worthlessness of the most medicines."
Benjamin Franklin

"150 people die every year from being hit by falling coconuts. Not to worry, drug makers are developing a vaccine."
~ Jim Carrey, Nov 20th 2009

Table of Contents

Introduction

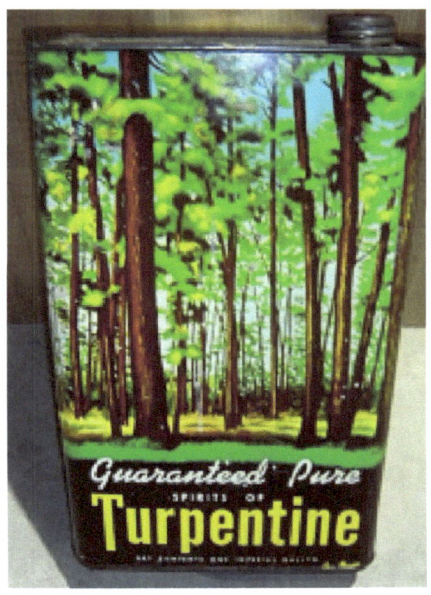

You will probably be just as surprised as I was upon learning that "turpentine" is yet another natural earth born product that is actually a natural medicinal healer. Turpentine is derived from the resin or sap of fir trees including, but not limited to Pine and Balsam Trees.

The scientific name for turpentine is *Pinus* and the family is Pinaceae which includes a number of species and varieties depending on origin. Common names for turpentine include gum turpentine, turpentine oil, turpentine balsam, spirit of turpentine, oil of turpentine, pine oil, pine gum, wood turpentine, terp and terpenic oil, among others.

Raw turpentine is a sticky resin and is brownish yellow in color. It dissolves sulphur, phosphorus and resins.

Turpentine's chemical formula is $C_{10}H_{16}$ and its boiling point is 155 – 185 C.

Raw turpentine is composed primarily of monoterpene hydrocarbons, the most prevalent of which are pinenes, camphene and 3-carene. Numerous other compounds are also present in all turpentine products, although in smaller quantities. The ratio between the different terpenes in turpentine varies according to its origin. For example, American turpentine contains a great deal more of both alpha and beta pinene over that of Swedish turpentine.

Turpentine has been used as a valuable medicinal remedy since the days of Hippocrates (460 BC – 370 BC) through to the turn of the twentieth century, when the Pharmaceutical industry took over medicine.

The purpose of this book is that of enlightenment, information and education.

Definitions of Turpentine

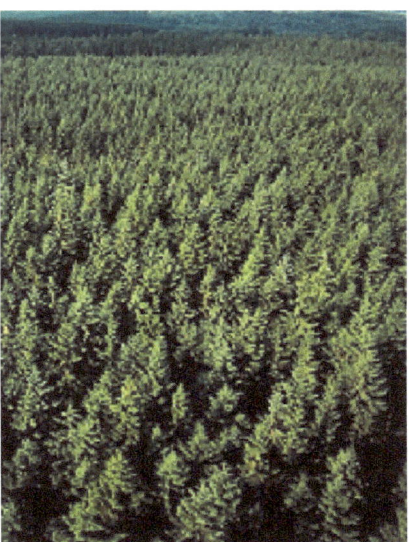

Pine forest in Sweden

The definition of turpentine, from the on-line Merriam-Webster dictionary, is as follows:

"1. a) a yellow to brown semifluid oleoresin obtained as an exudate from the terebinth

b) an **oleoresin** obtained from various conifers (as some pines and firs)

2. a) an essential oil obtained from turpentine by distillation and used especially as a solvent and thinner —called also gum turpentine

b) a similar oil obtained by distillation or carbonization of pinewood —called also wood turpentine."

As an FYI, the definition of **oleoresin** is: "a naturally occurring mixture of an oil and resin extracted from various plants, such as pine or balsam fir" http:// www.thefreedictionary.com.

From Concise Encyclopedia, turpentine is defined as:

"Any resinous exudate or extract from conifers, especially pines; now also commonly a term for its volatile fraction, oil (or spirits) of turpentine. Semifluid mixtures of organic compounds consisting of resins dissolved in a volatile oil, turpentine can be distilled (see distillation) into the volatile oil of turpentine and the nonvolatile rosin. The oil, a mixture of monoterpenes (see isoprenoid), chiefly Pinene, is a colorless, odorous, flammable liquid that does not mix with water but is a good solvent for many substances. Oil of turpentine is favored over petroleum solvents as an oil-paint thinner, varnish solvent, and brush cleaner. Its chief use is now as a raw material for resins, insecticides, oil additives, and synthetic pine oil and camphor and as a solvent."

Encyclopedia Britannica defines turpentine as the following:

"Turpentine, the resinous exudate or extract obtained from coniferous trees, particularly those of the genus Pinus (Pine). Turpentines are semifluid substances consisting of resins dissolved in a volatile oil; this mixture is separable by various distillation techniques into a volatile portion called oil (or spirit) of turpentine and a nonvolatile portion called rosin. Although the term turpentine originally referred to the whole oleoresinous exudate, it now commonly refers to its volatile turpentine fraction only, which has various uses in industry and the visual arts."

It is interesting to note that the above current definitions for turpentine omit the fact that it is and was historically used as a very potent healing remedy.

Traditional Native Medicine

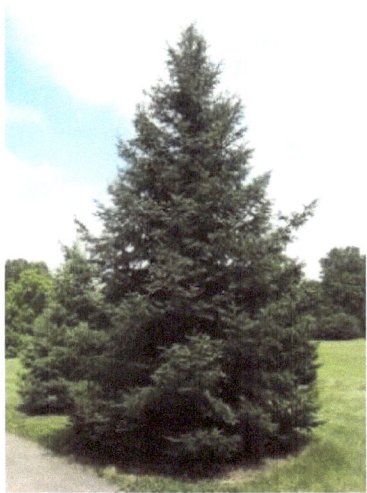

Balsam Fir Tree

The balsam fir tree has so much more to offer than just that of a cut down tree for use as the traditional Christmas tree in North America and abroad. Our Indigenous Forefathers, who knew all the secrets of the boreal forest, taught the French settlers to Canada the medicinal benefits that the balsam fir had to offer which included: a remedy against influenza and scurvy; an effective treatment for infections, insect bites, cuts, burns, and so much more. Almost every part of the tree provided some type of herbal remedy and the tree was essential in number of traditional native medicinal remedies.

Our Native Forefathers believed that medicine from the earth should never be altered since to do that, you thought of yourself as above the Creator. After all, Creation is perfect in the first place.

The resin of this fir tree was known as a very valuable commodity to the French settlers for industrial uses such as patching holes in their canoes.

The balsam fir resin became known as the "turpentine of Canada" as it proved to be an extraordinary product as a medicinal and industrial cure-all.

The boreal forest of Canada encompasses about one third of the land north of the 50th parallel. Other countries that are also blessed with a boreal forest include Russia, Scandinavian and Nordic countries such as Sweden, Finland and Norway. In Canada, the boreal forest covers almost sixty percent of her land.

Forest land in Canada, as with most land in Canada is "Crown land", meaning it belongs to the monarch (Queen of England).

Scientific Evidence vs. Empirical Evidence

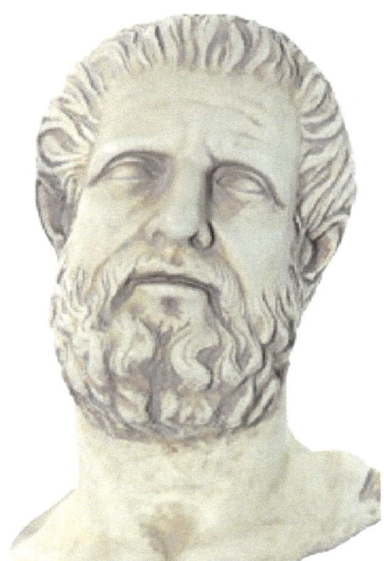

Hippocrates – 460 BC – 370 BC

Hippocrates is known as "the Father of Medicine". What Hippocrates did in terms of advancing medicine, is a true god sent. His systematic belief in documentation is known today as "clinical observation" or empirical evidence. Hippocrates, and other Greek Doctors, believed that observation of a patient was a major component in medical care. Hippocrates strived for a systematic documentation of the observation of what transpired within patient care. This man advanced medicine like no other. His strict protocol of "clinical observation" assisted all those that came after him. His protocol gave doctors a detailed method on what to do. By observing and recording patients on a day to day basis, allowed other doctors the ability of forecasting the development of illnesses and this continued into the future. Hippocrates was of the belief that all diseases had a natural cause (rather than a cause of an unknown source or origin). Hippocrates also believed that what doctors did needed to be kept separate and apart from that of Priests doings. It was believed by Priests that illnesses such as epilepsy were all an act of the Gods whereas Hippocrates believed that all and each disease was caused by a natural source. Hippocrates lived for eighty three years up to 377 BC!

The Natural Health Care Industry today is built on Hippocrates belief in that they utilize a method of healing based on what has consistently delivered a consistent result in the past. Such methods of natural healing become "generally accepted".

If not for the internet, we may have wrongly believed that Hippocrates was only another "philosopher", rather than a visionary and a doctor whom truly cared about patients and their health.

Evidence or science based medicine is now ingrained in our schools and history books as the only proven method despite that of empirical evidence that dates back thousands of years. Without science based evidence, we are told, one is unable to accept, adopt and/ or rely on anything but since anything but scientific based medicine considered unproven and unscientific. However, there is great fault with that basis of medicine in that it is not always able to be replicated a second or even third time. In other words, if we are to rely on the scientific method, should it not prove itself over and over again in scientific experiments? Unfortunately, if it was once proven, we are brainwashed into believing, it is scientific proof that the scientific based remedy is effective above all else.

The main flaw in science based medicine is that it is used as a "selective standard".

Evidence or science based medicine has become the norm over that of handed down observation or empirical based practices in medicine. I 1972, Archie Cochrane published "Effectiveness and Efficiency" which "described the lack of controlled trials supporting many practices that had previously been assumed to be effective." *(Cochrane A.L. (1972). Effectiveness and Efficiency: Random Reflections on Health Services. Nuffield Provincial Hospitals Trust.)*

As it stands today, anything other than scientific based medicine is considered "unproven" and therefore, not reliable, despite centuries of observed results. In actual fact, the scientific based argument seems to be just another tactic at eliminating competition.

History of Turpentine

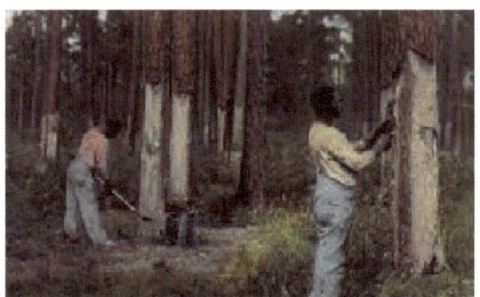

Turpentine industry – scraping pine trees in Florida

Britain's colonies in North America were instructed to produce pine tar and to also collect the gum from pine trees for future shipment to England. Beginning with the Bounty Act of 1705, when England was cut off from its Scandinavian supplies by Russia's invasion of Sweden-Finland, England was desperate for an alternate supply. By 1725, most of the tar and pitch used in England came from their new American colonies and continued until the American Revolution in 1776.

In 1840, Great Britain repealed her non-importation duties imposed on Naval Store with the United States which subsequently dramatically increased North Carolina's naval store production.

Before "trains, planes and automobiles", there were naval stores, or stores that "stored" things for later use in the building and maintenance of ships. By the end of the colonial period, naval stores included everything needed in ship building including tar, pitch and turpentine – all of which were manufactured from pine trees.

Pine trees produce a gummy, sticky sap and pine resin is able to produce a sticky mess that is quite a chore to remove from your fingers and hands. However, that same sap is what protects the tree and this sap is also capable of protecting other wood from the hazards of weather, including weather proofing the wooden hulls of ships.

Following is a definition of extracts produced from pine tree sap:

Tar: a dark, thick, sticky liquid that is produced from burning pine branches and logs in kilns. Tar kept ropes and sail rigging from decaying.

Pitch: a product obtained from boiling tar in order to concentrate it. In colonial times, pitch was used to make wooden ships waterproof (thereby preventing leakage) just by painting this product onto the bottom of ships.

Turpentine: is "distilled" from the gum that pine trees secrete. Turpentine, as a natural secretion from pine trees, has a long history in medicine. However, beginning in the nineteenth century, it began its use as a paint thinner and remover.

Rosin: a solid substance obtained from the by-product after distilling turpentine. It is the solid material left behind after distilling turpentine. Rosin was used in making varnishes, soaps, adhesives and numerous other products.

Early in the eighteenth century, Britain was anxious for naval supplies since they had used up their local sources of trees. To encourage American naval stores, the British Parliament passed a law in 1705 that dictated a requirement for the British Navy to pay inflated prices for tar, pitch, turpentine, rosin, hemp and masts from the British colonies.

In the book "Looking for Longleaf: The Rise and Fall of an American Forest", the author, Lawrence Earley, noted that without tar, pitch, turpentine and rosin along with the access to the forests from which they came, Britain's military and commercial shipping fleets would have otherwise been useless and her ambitions fruitless."

The turpentine camps of pre and post-civil war, in order to meet Britain's naval store demands, destroyed not only whole forests of trees, it also destroyed hundreds of men most of whom were African Americans. These camps were said to be "slavery under a new name". The turpentine industry after the end of the Civil War, contained one of the harshest and most brutal systems of labor to ever function due to a system of debt bondage and the abuse of the penal system's "leasing of prisoners", most of whom were African Americans.

In his 1821 book *"The Medical Repository"* by Dr. Samuel Osborn, he states the following about turpentine: "It is not to be expected that any medicine will operate more powerfully than this does …".

The 1939 book "The Modern Home Physician" states, "Turpentine is sometimes used in half ounce doses, with an equal quantity of castor oil, as a means of killing and dislodging tapeworms."

Turpentine has a long history of use as a paint solvent; however this use has dwindled considerably in favor of less expensive petroleum solvents. In fact, turpentine manufactured from petroleum solvents became known as mineral turpentine to distinguish it from the natural turpentine extracted from wood.

In recent years, a renewed interest in traditional methods was thought to have created a comeback for natural turpentine but it is marginal relative to the quantity of petroleum solvents that dominate most industries today.

Pinene – the Essence of Turpentine

TERPENE	BENEFIT	AROMA
Pinene Also found in pine needles	Anti-inflamatory Anti-bacterial Bronchodilator Aids memory	Pine Earth

Turpentine is a complex mixture of terpenes, the most volatile of which are alpha and beta pinene. These two terpenes are the odorous compounds that are emitted by many trees, shrubs, flowers grasses, weeds and cannabis.

The chemical substance - alpha-pinene, is a major component in a number of essential oils (concentrated essence of plant material). Alpha-pinene is known as a terpene, which is one of the most common compounds found in nature and is most prevalent in the coniferous pine tree. Alpha-pinene is notable for its highly effective anti-inflammatory and antimicrobial properties.

Recent research has shown that the presence of a greater content of alpha pinene over beta-pinene is effective in fighting pathogenic bacteria and all kinds of fungi and parasites including Candida albicans and E-coli. Studies have shown that alpha-pinene is able to eliminate the micro-organisms or greatly inhibit their growth plus halt their metabolism. Alpha-pinene is also an effective insecticide especially against mosquitoes. It is also noted as effective in preventing bacteria causing jaw infections and periodontist disease. Additionally, alpha-pinene is effective as an inhibitor against breast cancer and has impressive antioxidative abilities.

Beta-pinene usually accompanies a-pinene in lower quantities and together with a-pinene is anti-tumorous. When a and b pinenes are the major constituents in this and other essential oils, they are an effective anti-inflammatory and also have an analgesic effect.

United States Pharmacopeia (USP)

The USP, in 1913, defined turpentine oil as follows:

"Oleum Terebinthinae.—Oil Of Turpentine, U. S. P.

A volatile oil recently distilled from turpentine.

Properties: Oil of turpentine occurs as a thin colorless liquid, having a characteristic odor and taste, both of which become stronger and less pleasant by age and exposure to air. Oil of turpentine is practically insoluble in water, but freely soluble in alcohol (1:3), and in all proportions of oil. For internal use the rectified oil of turpentine (Oleum Terebinthinae Rectiflcatum) should be used.

Action and Uses: Turpentine is antiseptic, anthelmintic and diuretic. Applied externally it is rubefacient and counterirritant.

Turpentine has been used as an expectorant in cases of bronchitis characterized by free secretion. For this purpose it is now generally replaced by terpin hydrate. It is also given for the relief of flatulence and a small amount (from ½ to 1 teaspoonful) may he added to enemas to increase their effectiveness.

Turpentine has been thought to be efficient in cases of internal hemorrhages, but this opinion is not well founded.

Dosage: 1 c.c. or 15 minims. It may be administered in the form of emulsion or in capsules."

The first edition of the **Merck Manual**, published in 1899, states that "turpentine therapy is effective for a wide range of conditions including gonorrhea, meningitis, arthritis, abdominal difficulties and lung disease." However, the more recent 1999 *Merck Manual* mentions only the dire effects of turpentine poisoning with destruction of the kidneys and lungs.

Phytotherapy of Turpentine

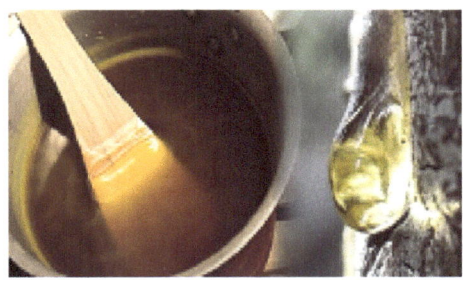

For thousands of years prior to the twentieth century, people would strip the bark from the pine tree and puncture the tree trunk as a way to collect droplets of the tree's resin. The resin collected was then distilled with water and became known as turpentine. Turpentine is rich in both alpha and beta pinenes and is used in a number of home remedies. When diluted in milk, wine or water, the concoction was used for respiratory problems and was also noted as an effective expectorant. In addition, any one of the aforementioned concoctions was used both internally and externally as an effective cure for any of a number of parasitic infections. Alpha-pinene or a-pinene is also an effective broad spectrum antibiotic. *(NissenL, Zatta A, Stefanini I, Grandi S, Sgorbati B, Biavati B , et al. (2010))*

Hippocrates and other doctors of his era, prescribed turpentine for its properties against lung disease and biliary stones (gallbladder and/ or kidney stones). In the early nineteenth century in France, turpentine was prescribed for excessive mucus or bladder inflammation. In Germany, Slovenia and Poland, turpentine was prescribed for the following severe conditions: severe pain that resulted from a damaged nerve; rheumatism, lower back pain, kidney inflammation; constipation and mercury poisoning. These prescribing doctors recognized that turpentine was an effective booster at an average dose but would be paralyzing at high doses.

Modern Phytotherapy of turpentine describes the following properties: ant parasitic, external disinfectant, analgesic, balsamic (soften or reduce mucus), hemostasis (ability to stop bleeding), antispasmodic, diuretic, ant rheumatic, deworming, antidote for poisoning caused by phosphorus, reduces bronchial secretion and other chronic obstructive bronchitis.

Mixing 1 tsp of turpentine in 4 oz. of honey is an effective oral remedy for inflammation, breathing, fungus, viral, bacterial and as an antioxidant.

Mixing 1 oz. of turpentine with 5 ox of peanut oil is effective when topically applied to damaged or congested skin, open wounds, festering infections, stiff joints and when applied topically to the bronchial area, is able to penetrate and break down lung infections.

When mixed with olive oil or coconut oil in a ratio of 2 parts oil to 1 part turpentine, it is effective at removing narcotic poisoning due to an enema effect.

Turpentine can cause an increased secretion of urine and relieve back pains that result from backed up kidneys.

Turpentine and the Chemical Industry

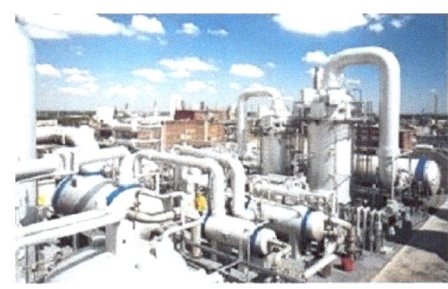

In the early twentieth century, the use of turpentine in pharmaceuticals and chemicals was relatively minor. However, by the 1940's, the consumption of turpentine by these industries rose exponentially and became quite significant. The reason for this increase was due to the rise in production of synthetic camphor in which turpentine plays a major role. The first large scale production of synthetic camphor in the US began with a DuPont plant in 1932. By 1946, the plastic industry's demand for sufficient quantities of synthetic camphor was met and was 5,000,000 pounds per year.

According to current literature, the largest use for turpentine in the past was as a paint and varnish solvent, thinner and brush cleaner. Turpentine was also added to many cleaning and sanitary products due to its antiseptic properties and its pine scent. Turpentine was also found in varnishes, floor and furniture waxes and polishes, pottery and ceramic coatings, artist paints and paint brush cleaners. It was also used in hair products, printing and as a metal cleaner. Today however, less costly products have replaced the use of turpentine in paints.

Today, the major use of turpentine is as a raw material in the chemical industry. Compounds extracted from turpentine are used for tires, plastics, adhesives, flavors, fragrances, makeup, paints and medicine.

Turpentine oil is classified according to the way it is produced.

Sulfate turpentine, which is largely used in the chemical industry, is obtained as a by-product in the process of cooking wood pulp in the manufacture of paper. It is this product that poses a danger to our health due to the chemical content thanks to the chemical industry.

Mineral turpentine is a petroleum distillate used to replace real turpentine and is very different chemically.

Wood turpentine is obtained from the process of steam distillation of dead, shredded bits of pine wood.

Gum turpentine is derived from the natural process of tapping the live tree. This type of turpentine is what was historically used as a medicinal cure-all. Today, the pharmaceutical and chemical industries control turpentine in North America.

Conclusion

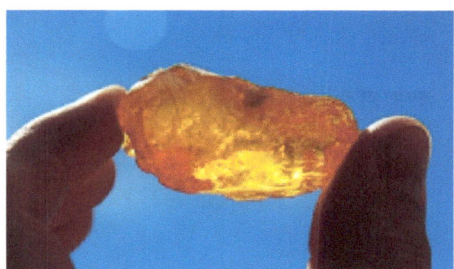

Alpha-pinene

The essential oil of turpentine and its two major pinene terpenes, have very effective natural healing properties along with other medicinal benefits. As a natural product from various species of pine trees, it poses no hazard when taken in small doses. The number of benefits this ancient cure-all was known for is a much needed resource to our health and well-being.

Over the course of many years, several different systems of tapping have evolved. Regardless to how it is performed, tapping should be carefully conducted in a way to avoid damage to the tree.

As a natural cure-all, is it any wonder that we have been taught (by Big Pharma no less) that this product is hazard to our health?

Noteworthy

Some of the listings for Terebinth (Turpentine)

Internal Uses for Terebinth – Turpenine

Modifies tracheo-bronchial secretions
Haemostatic (slows down or stops bleeding)
Diuretic
Antirheumatic
Antidote to Phosphorus Poisoning

Indications
Chronic and Fetid Bronchitis
Pulmonary TB (lung TB)

Leucorrhia (vaginal discharge)
Haemorrhage (intestinal-pulmonary-uterine-haempohilia-nose bleeds)
Oliguria (diuretic like effect)
Rheumatism (painful body)
Flatulence
Intestinal Parasites (especially worms)
Epilepsy
Phosporus Antidote

Internal Uses for Terebinth – Turpenine

Genitor-Urinary Antiseptic (used as a douche as well injectable
Dissolves Gallstones
Antispasmodic
Vermifuge (removes worms and parasites

Indications
Urinary and Renal Infections-cystitis urethritis (inflammation of the urethra)
Puerperal Fever-(infection of the uterus after birth)
Gallstones
Dropsy (excess water retention of organs or tissue)
Spasms (Colitis-whopping Cough)
Migraine
Chronic Constipation

External Uses For Terebinth-Turpentine-

Parasiticide
Revulsive (counter irritant or antidotal)

USES
Rheumatism-Gout-Neuralgia-Sciatica
Scabies or Lice
Puerporal Infections (bleeding under the skin –purple spots)

External Uses For Terebinth-Turpentine-

Analgesic
Antiseptic

USES
Atonic wounds(a slow healing wound or a damaged or weakened muscle-
Sores and Gangrescous wounds
Leucorrhea

From Toney Pantalleresco's "Herbs Plus Bead Works" You Tube Channel

Closing Remarks

"It's painful not to be treated as an equal. You have to be strong to walk through the storm. It's like being a bridge between two worlds. If this is the case, all I ask is for people to wash their feet before they try to walk on me."

Alanis Obomsawin

"Christopher Columbus is a symbol, not of a man, but of imperialism. Imperialism and colonialism are not something that happened decades ago or generations ago, but they are still happening now with the exploitation of people."

John Mohawk

About The Author

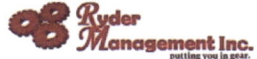

Ryder Management Inc. (Rydermgt or RMI) is a Canadian Controlled Private Corporation (CCPC) based in London, ON Canada. As an "umbrella" organization, RMI brings together a group of authors whom are professionals in their respective fields and are writing with the primary goal of providing books that educate, comfort and offer assurance that natural remedies do exist and are an effective and safe way to regain, obtain and maintain health.

www.ingramcontent.com/pod-product-compliance
Lightning Source LLC
Chambersburg PA
CBHW050925290526
45792CB00002B/893